rivers' walk

Presented by

The Memphis Oral School for the Deaf
and
Innovo Publishing LLC

Story courtesy of Dr. Nathalie Johnson, Audiologist at MOSD
Illustrations & Publishing Services courtesy of Innovo Publishing LLC

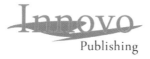

Innovo
Publishing

Published by
Innovo Publishing LLC
www.innovopublishing.com
1-888-546-2111

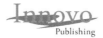

Providing Full-Service Publishing Services for
Christian Authors, Artists & Organizations: Hardbacks, Paperbacks,
eBooks, Audiobooks, Music & Videos.

RIVER'S WALK

ISBN 13: 978-1-936076-35-2
ISBN 10: 1-936076-35-7

Cover Design & Interior Layout: Innovo Publishing LLC

Printed in the United States of America
U.S. Printing History
First Edition: August 2010

DEDICATION AND ACKNOWLEDGMENT

For more than 50 years, the Memphis Oral School for the Deaf (MOSD) has faithfully served our community and provided hope to countless children and their families by empowering deaf children to listen, learn, and talk. In recognition of MOSD's mission and community service, Innovo Publishing is pleased to donate our services and to dedicate this book to the Memphis Oral School for the Deaf—and to the children and families whom it serves.

Dr. Bart Dahmer
Principal & Managing Partner
Innovo Publishing LLC

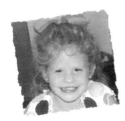

This story was inspired by a very real and very special little girl named Rivers (left). Her zest for life and vibrant character bring a smile to the faces of everyone she meets. Read more about Rivers and her experience with MOSD at the end of this book.

In memory of Gayble Young Moss

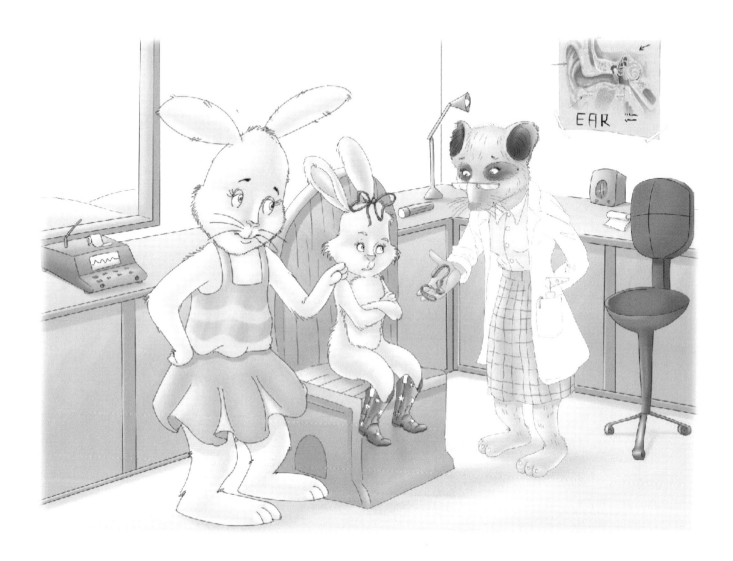

Rivers was a happy, light-hearted little bunny. But today she was neither happy nor light-hearted. Her mother had taken her to the audiologist to pick up her new hearing aids. Rivers had made it very clear that she did NOT want hearing aids. But here they were, nonetheless.

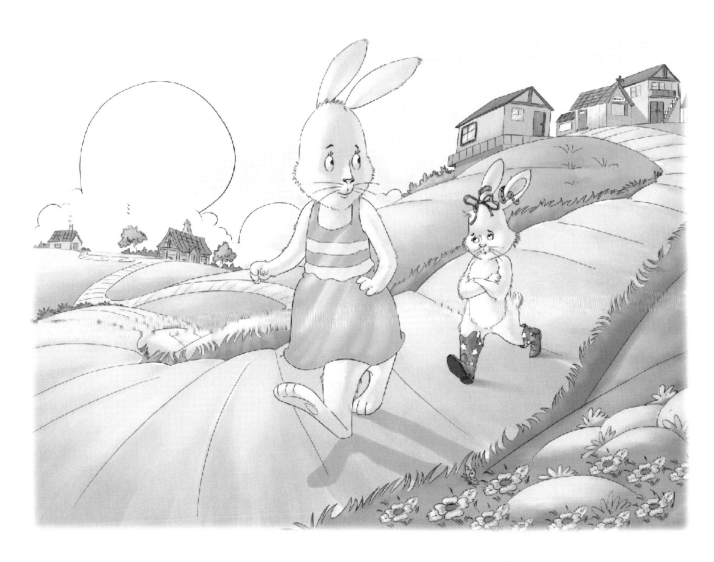

Rivers did not say a word the whole way home.

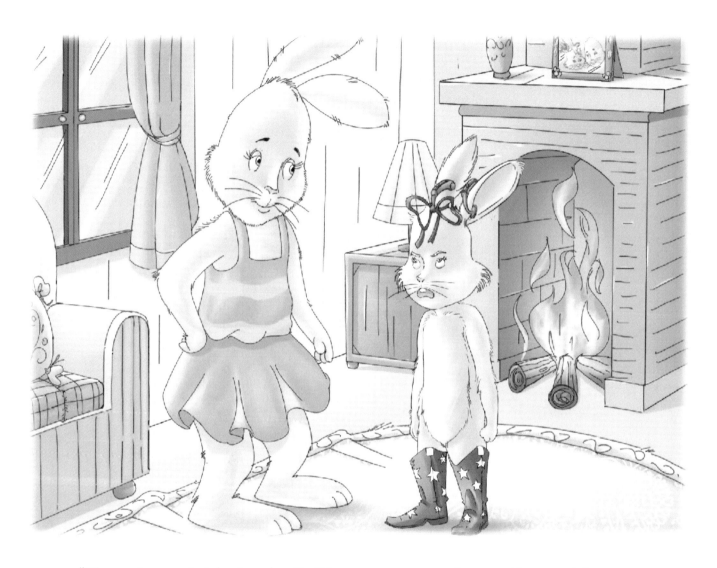

"I'm going outside to play!" Rivers announced once they got home.

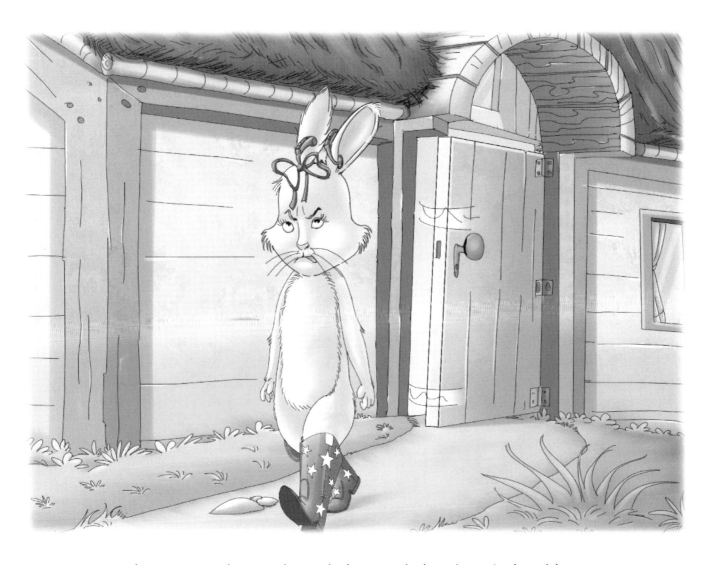

She stomped outside and slammed the door behind her.

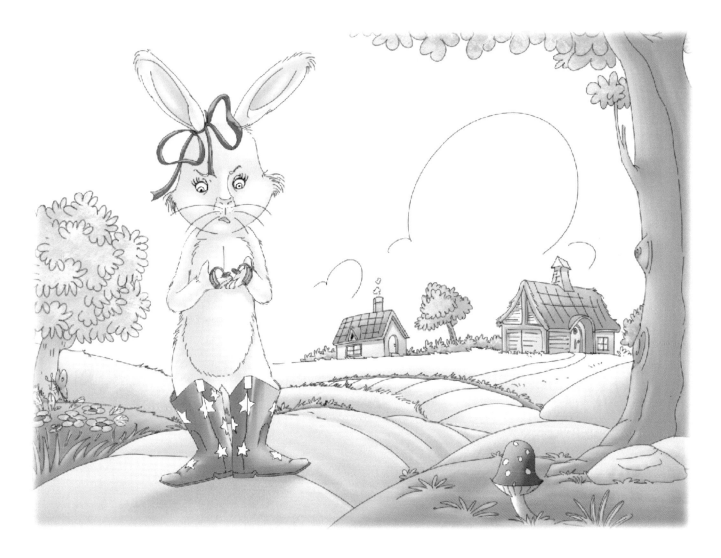

Rivers thought about her new hearing aids. They felt funny in her ears.
They felt itchy in her ears. She took them out to take a closer look. She did
not like them one bit.

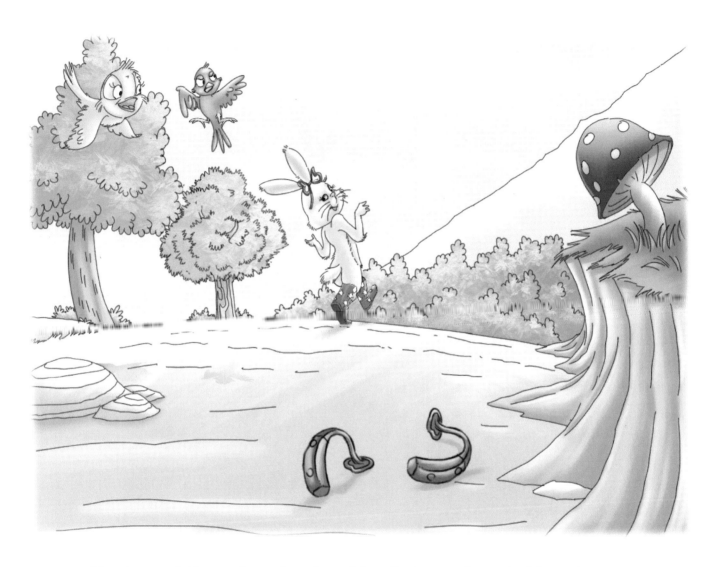

She tossed them down by the side of the path and skipped away.

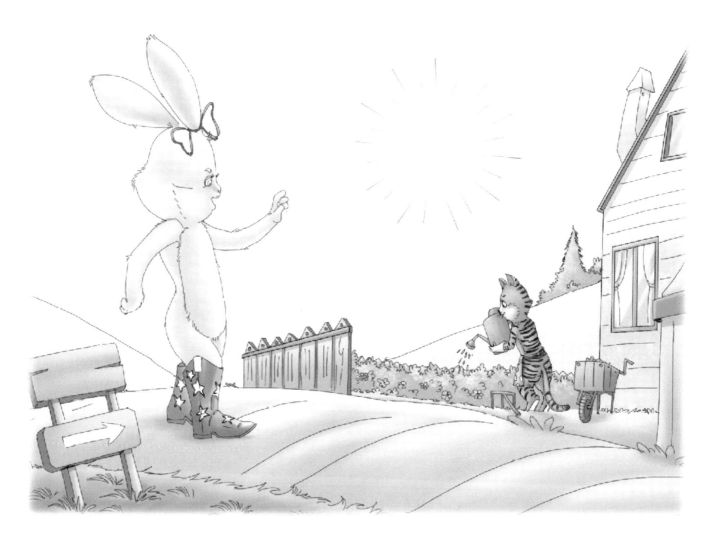

As she skipped along, she could feel the sunshine on her soft bunny fur. "What a wonderful day for dancing," she thought. Just then she saw her friend Louise.

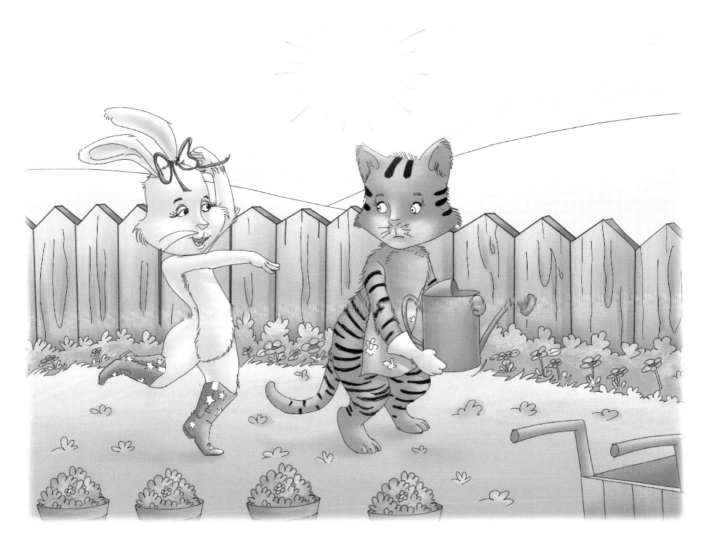

"Louise", called Rivers. "Do you want to dance with me?" But Louise did not answer. Perhaps she did not hear her. "LOUISE...DO YOU WANT TO DANCE WITH ME?" Rivers said. Again, Louise did not answer. Feeling slightly disappointed, Rivers skipped away down the path.

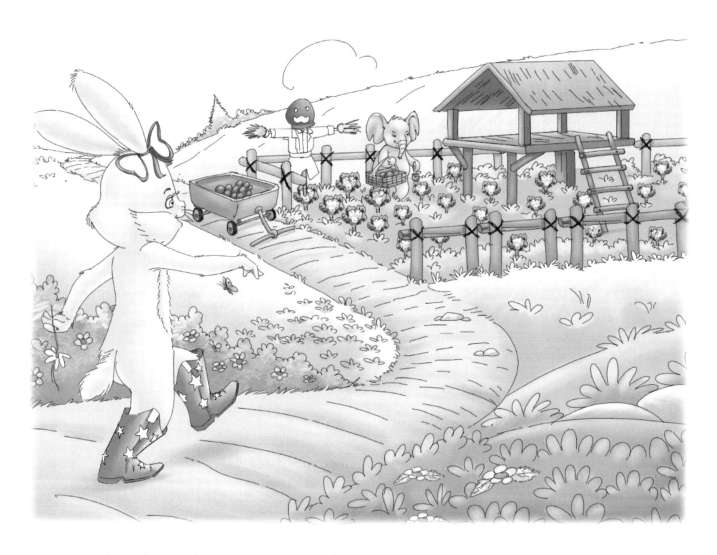

As she skipped along, she could smell the sweet flowers with her tiny bunny nose. "What a wonderful day for singing," she thought. Just then she saw her friend Claire.

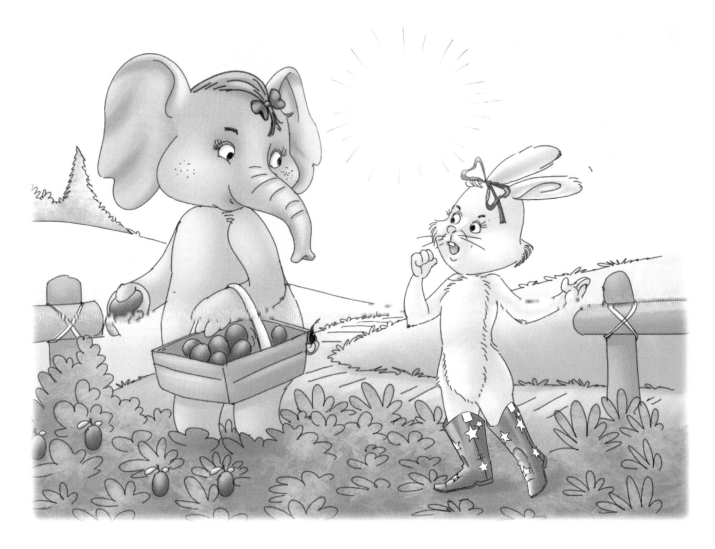

"Claire," called Rivers. "Do you want to sing with me?" But Claire did not answer. Perhaps she did not hear her. "CLAIRE...DO YOU WANT TO SING WITH ME?" Rivers said. Again, Claire did not answer. Feeling even more disappointed, Rivers slowly skipped away down the path.

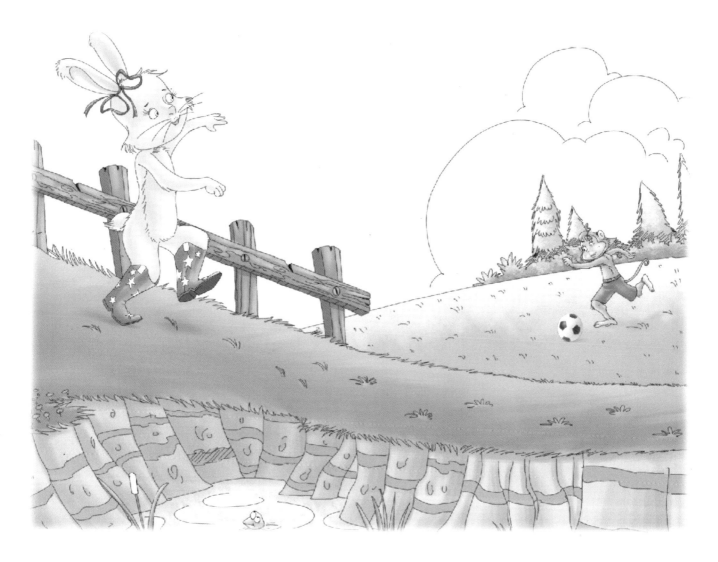

As she skipped along, Rivers could see the clouds floating in the sky with her big bunny eyes. "What a wonderful day for playing," she thought. Just then she saw her friend Kate.

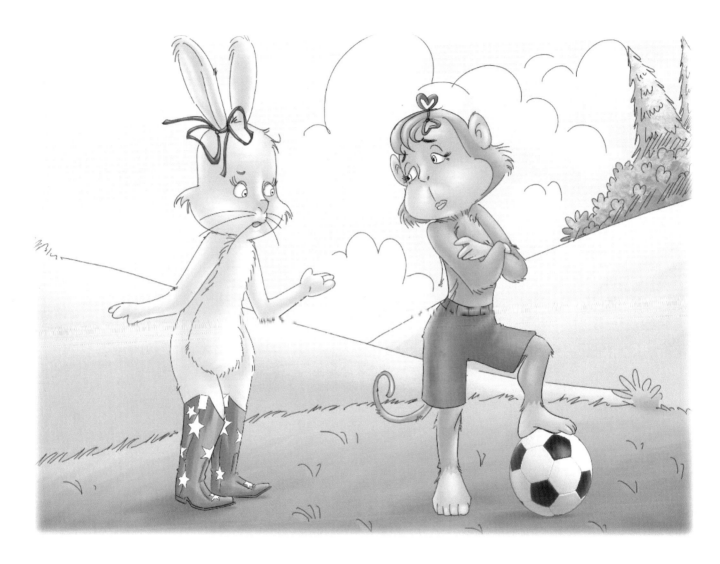

"Kate", called Rivers. "Do you want to play with me?" But Kate did not answer. Perhaps she did not hear her. "KATE...DO YOU WANT TO PLAY WITH ME?" Rivers said. Again, Kate did not answer. Feeling even more disappointed, Rivers hung her head and slowly walked down the path.

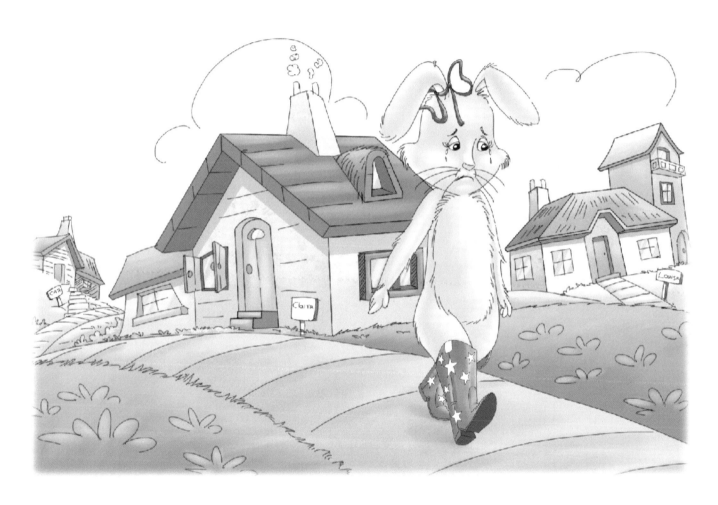

She could not understand why her friends did not want to dance or sing or play. Did they not think she *could*? Rivers *could* dance. She *could* sing. She *could* play. She hung her head low and walked back towards her house.

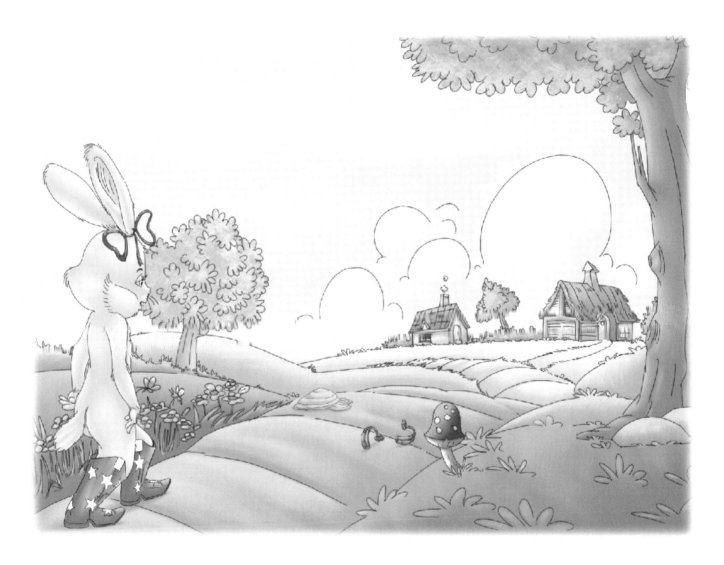

      As she got closer to her house, Rivers saw something sparkly on the side of the path. It was her hearing aids. She picked them up and placed them in her paw. This time, they did not look so bad. They were actually quite sparkly and glittery.

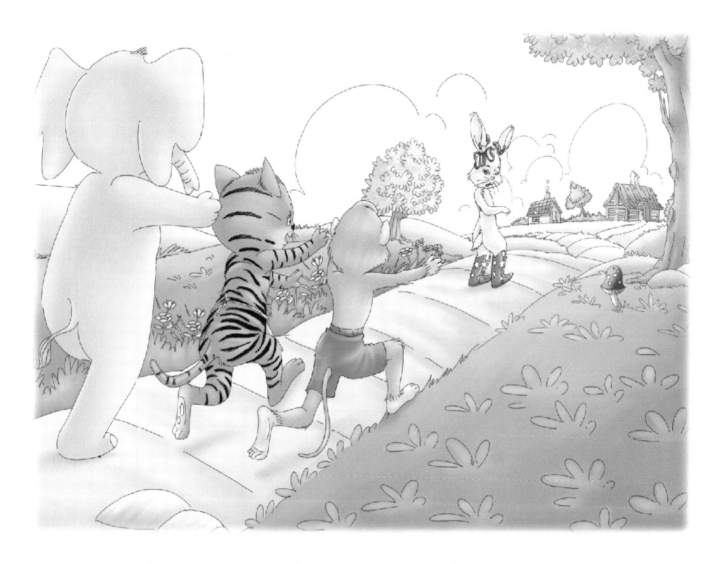

She slowly put them back in her ears. This time, they were not so scratchy. This time, they were not so itchy. Then something amazing happened. She could hear her friends calling her name.

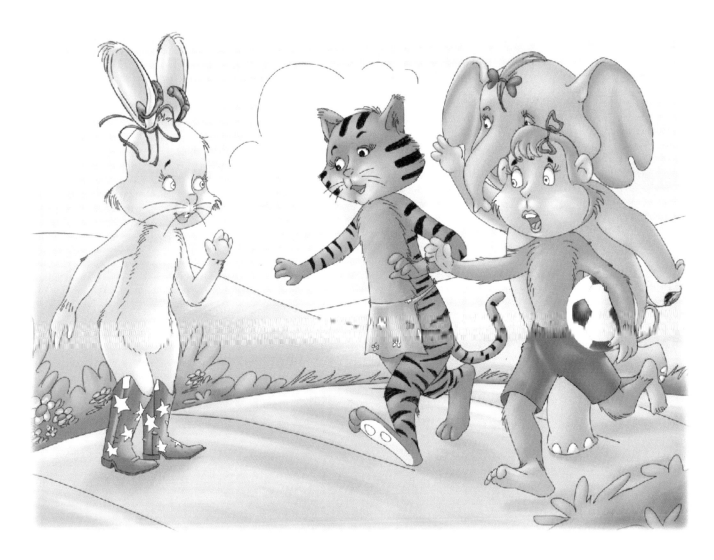

"RIVERS!" "RIVERS!" "RIVERS!" they were shouting. Louise *did* want to dance. Claire *did* want to sing. Kate *did* want to play. They had been trying to tell her all along. But without her hearing aids on, Rivers had not heard them.

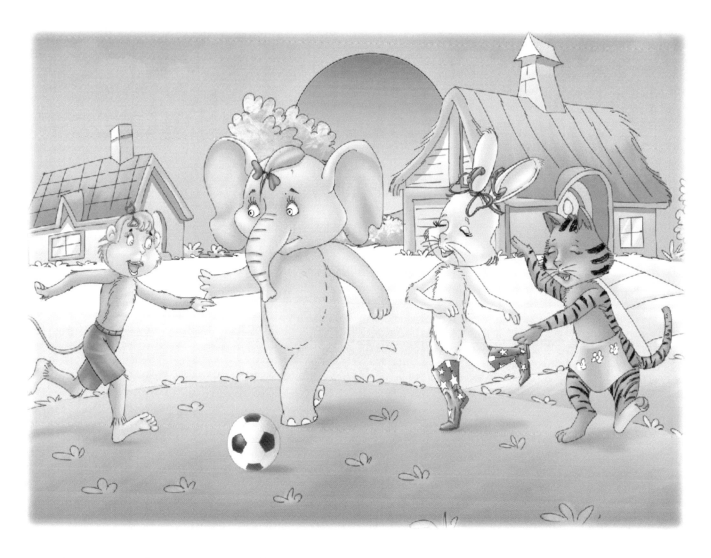

Rivers and Louise and Claire and Kate danced and sang and played until the hot sun that had felt so warm on Rivers' soft bunny fur sank deep down out of the sky.

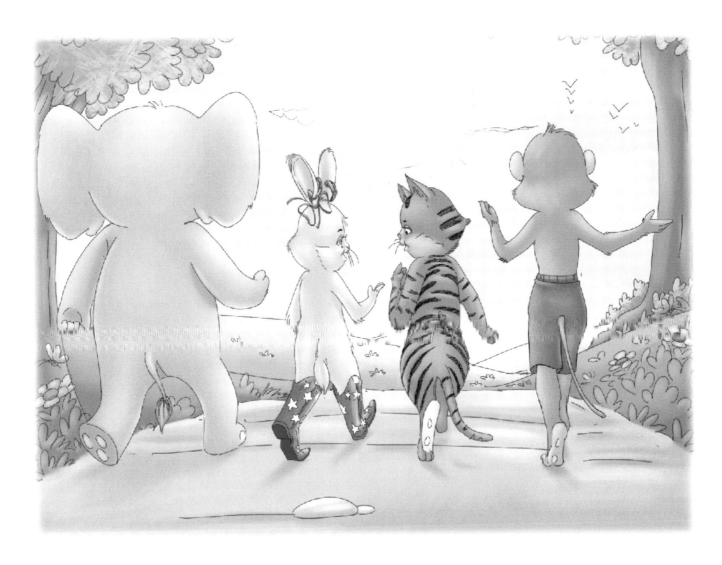

From that day on, Rivers wore her hearing aids every day and never complained about them again.

MEET THE "REAL-LIFE" RIVERS

The "real-life" Rivers is a sassy, talkative five-year-old who lives in Oxford, Mississippi, with her mom, dad, and two brothers. When Rivers was only three weeks old, she was diagnosed with profound hearing loss and was immediately fitted with hearing aids. It was later determined that she would gain more benefit from cochlear implants because of her profound loss. The first implantation was performed when Rivers was fourteen months old; the second, when she was three years old.

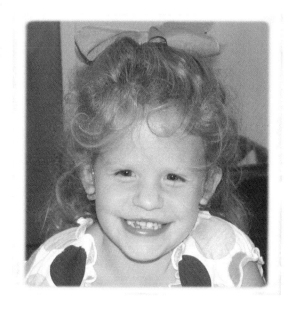

In order to give her every available tool to ensure her success, Rivers was enrolled at the Memphis Oral School for the Deaf when she was two. She has attended MOSD for three years, and her speech and language skills have exploded!

The Memphis Oral School for the Deaf makes life-changing miracles happen for hundreds of special children just like Rivers.

ABOUT THE AUTHOR

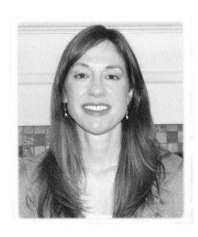

Dr. Nathalie Johnson received her undergraduate degree in Speech and Hearing Sciences from Indiana University, her masters degree in Audiology from the University of Memphis, and recently her doctorate in Audiology from the Arizona School of Health Sciences. She has dedicated the last 15 years of her professional career to the children and families at The Memphis Oral School for the Deaf, where she is head of the family training program entitled *Sound Beginnings*. Dr. Johnson shares the vision of The Memphis Oral School for the Deaf where every day is an opportunity to give the gift of sound and to empower deaf children to listen, learn, and talk.

ABOUT MOSD

Located in the Memphis community for more than fifty years and serving families from all over the Mid-South, The Memphis Oral School for the Deaf works to empower deaf children to listen, learn, and talk. At MOSD, no sign language is used. Instead, it employs speech and language therapies and audiological services, in conjunction with preschool classes, to help profoundly deaf and hard-of-hearing children ages birth to six years old. These specialized techniques help the children develop the necessary listening and spoken language skills to become a part of, rather than apart from, a world of sound. Find out more at www.MOSDkids.org.

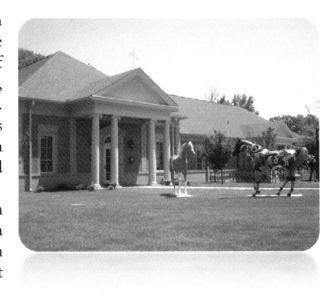

ABOUT INNOVO PUBLISHING LLC

Innovo Publishing LLC is a full-service Christian publishing company serving the Christian and wholesome markets. Innovo creates, distributes, and markets quality books, eBooks, audiobooks, music, and videos through traditional and innovative publishing models and services. Innovo provides distribution, marketing, and automated order fulfillment through a network of thousands of physical and online wholesalers, retailers, bookstores, music stores, schools, and libraries worldwide. Innovo provides a unique combination of traditional publishing, co-publishing, and independent (self) publishing arrangements that allow authors, artists, and organizations to accomplish their personal, organizational, and philanthropic publishing goals. Visit Innovo Publishing's web site at www.innovopublishing.com or email Innovo at info@innovopublishing.com.

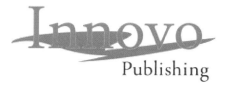

LaVergne, TN USA
08 October 2010
199950LV00002B